RAPID WEIGHT LOSS HYPNOSIS

A Complete Guide to Weight Loss And Eat Healthy Through Hypnosis, Meditation, Affirmations, And Motivation

Brenda Ewing

© Copyright 2021 Brenda Ewing

Rapid Weight Loss Hypnosis

© Copyright 2021 Brenda Ewing All rights reserved.

Written by Brenda Ewing

First Edition

Table of Contents

Introduction

While brainwashing is a notable type of mind control that numerous individuals have about, hypnosis is additionally a significant sort that ought to be thought of.

Generally, the individuals who know about it think about it from watching stage shows of members doing silly acts. While this is a sort of hypnosis, there is much more to it. This part is going to focus more on it as a type of mind control.

To begin with, what is the meaning of hypnosis? As indicated condition by specialists, cognizance consideration alongside hypnosis is viewed that includes the engaged and the diminished fringe mindfulness that is described by the member's expanded ability to react to recommendations that are given.

This implies the member will enter an alternate perspective and will be substantially more defenseless to following the recommendations that are given by the trance inducer. It is broadly perceived that two hypothesis bunches help to depict what's going on during the hypnosis time frame.

The first is the changing state hypothesis. The individuals who follow this hypothesis see that hypnosis resembles a daze or a perspective that is adjusted where the member will see that their mindfulness is, to some degree, not quite the same as what they would see in their common cognizant state. The other hypothesis is non-state speculations. The individuals who follow this hypothesis don't believe that the individuals who experience hypnosis are going into various conditions of awareness. Or maybe, the member is working with the subliminal specialist to enter a sort of inventive job authorization.

While in hypnosis, the member is thought to have more fixation and center that couples together with another capacity to focus on a particular memory or thought strongly.

During this procedure, the member is likewise ready to shut out different sources that may be diverting to them.

The mesmerizing subjects are thought to demonstrate an increased capacity to react to recommendations that are given to them, particularly when these proposals originate from the subliminal specialist.

The procedure that is utilized to put the member into hypnosis is knitted hypnotic enlistment and will include a progression of proposals and guidelines that are utilized as a kind of warm-up.

There is a wide range of musings that are raised by specialists with regards to what the meaning of hypnosis is.

The wide assortment of these definitions originates from the way that there are simply such huge numbers of various conditions that accompany hypnosis, and nobody individual has a similar encounter when they are experiencing it.

Some various perspectives and articulations have been made about hypnosis. A few people accept that hypnosis is genuine and are suspicious that the legislature and others around them will attempt to control their minds.

Others don't have faith in hypnosis at all and feel that it is only skillful deception. No doubt, the possibility of hypnosis as mind control falls someplace in the center.

There are three phases of hypnosis that are perceived by the mental network. These three phases incorporate acceptance, recommendation, and defenselessness.

Every one of them is critical to the hypnosis procedure and will be talked about further underneath.

Induction

The principal phase of hypnosis is induction. Before the member experiences the full hypnosis, they will be acquainted with the hypnotic enlistment method.

For a long time, this was believed to be the strategy used to place the subject into their hypnotic stupor. However, that definition has changed some in current occasions.

A portion of the non-state scholars has seen this stage somewhat in an unexpected way. Rather they consider this to be as the strategy to elevate the

Members' desires for what will occur, characterizing the job that they will play, standing out enough to be noticed to center the correct way, and any of the different advances that are required to lead the member into the correct heading for hypnosis.

There are a few induction procedures that can be utilized during hypnosis. The most notable and compelling strategies are Braid's "eye obsession" method or "Braidism."

There is a methodology, including many varieties of this the Stanford Hypnotic Susceptibility Scale (SHSS). This scale is the most utilized instrument to examine in the field of hypnosis.

To utilize the Braid enlistment procedures, you should follow several means. The first is to take any object that you can find that is brilliant, for example, a watch case, and hold it between the centers, fore, and thumb fingers on the left hand.

You will need to hold this item around 8—15 crawls from the eyes of the member.

Hold the item someplace over the brow, so it creates a ton of strain on the eyelids and eyes during the procedure with the goal that the member can keep up a fixed gaze on the article consistently. The trance inducer should then disclose to the member that they should focus their eyes consistently on the article.

The patient will likewise need to concentrate their mind on that specific item. They ought not to be permitted to consider different things or let their minds and eyes meander or, in all likelihood, the procedure won't be effective.

A little while later, the member's eyes will start to enlarge. With somewhat more time, the member will start to accept a wavy movement.

If the member automatically shuts their eyelids when the center and forefingers of the correct hand are conveyed from the eyes to the item, at that point, they are in a stupor.

If not, at that point, the member should start once more; make a point to tell the member that they are to permit their eyes to close once the fingers are conveyed in a comparable movement back towards the eyes once more. This will get the patient to go into the adjusted perspective that is knaps hypnosis.

While Braid remained by his method, he acknowledged that utilizing the acceptance procedure of hypnosis isn't constantly fundamental for each case.

Analysts on current occasions have typically discovered that the acceptance strategy isn't as essential with the impacts of hypnotic recommendation as recently suspected.

After some time, different other options and varieties of the first hypnotic acceptance procedure have been created, even though the Braid strategy is as yet thought about the best.

Recommendation

Present-day sleep induction utilizes a variety of proposal shapes to be fruitful, for example, representations, implications, roundabout or non-verbal recommendations, direct verbal proposals, and different metaphors and recommendations that are non-verbal.

A portion of the non-verbal proposals that might be utilized during the recommendation stage would incorporate physical manipulation, voice tonality, and mental symbolism.

One of the qualifications that are made in the kinds of recommendation that can be offered to the member incorporates those proposals that are conveyed with consent and those that progressively tyrant in the way.

Something that must be considered concerning hypnosis is the contrast between the oblivious and the cognizant mind.

There are a few trance specialists who see the phase of the proposal as a method of conveying that is guided generally to the cognizant mind of the subject.

Others in the field will see it the other way; they see the correspondence happening between the operator and the subconscious or oblivious mind.

They accepted that the recommendations were being tended to directly to the conscious piece of the subject's mind, as opposed to the oblivious part.

Braid goes further and characterizes the demonstration of trance induction as the engaged consideration upon the proposal or the predominant thought.

The fear of a great many people that subliminal specialists will have the option to get into their oblivious and cause them to do and think things outside their ability to control is inconceivable as per the individuals who follow this line of reasoning.

The idea of the mind has a determinant of the various additionally been the originations about the recommendation. The individuals who accepted that the reactions given are through the oblivious mind, for example, on account of Milton

Erickson, raise the instances of utilizing aberrant recommendations.

Huge numbers of these aberrant proposals, for example, stories or representations, will shroud their expected importance to cover it from the cognizant mind of the subject.

The subconscious recommendation is a type of hypnosis that depends on the hypothesis of the oblivious mind.

If the oblivious mind were not being utilized in hypnosis, this sort of recommendation would not be conceivable.

The contrasts between the two gatherings are genuinely simple to perceive; the individuals who accept that the recommendations will go fundamentally to the cognizant mind will utilize direct verbal guidelines and proposals while the individuals who accept the proposals will go essentially to the oblivious mind will utilize stories and analogies with concealed implications.

The member should have the option to concentrate on one article or thought. This permits them to be driven toward the path that is required to go into the hypnotic state.

When the recommendation stage has been finished effectively, the member will, at that point, have the option to move into the third stage, powerlessness.

Powerlessness After some time, it has been seen that individuals will respond contrastingly to hypnosis. A few people find that they can fall into a hypnotic stupor reasonably effectively and don't need to invest a lot of energy into the procedure by any means.

Others may find that they can get into the hypnotic daze, however, simply after a drawn-out timeframe and with some exertion. Still, others will find that they can't get into the hypnotic stupor, and significantly after proceeding with endeavors, won't arrive at their objectives. One thing that specialists have discovered intriguing about the weakness of various members is that this factor stays steady.

If you have had the option to get into a hypnotic perspective effectively, you are probably going to be on a similar path for an incredible remainder.

Then again, if you have consistently experienced issues in arriving at the hypnotic state and have never been entranced, at that point, almost certainly, you never will.

There have been a few distinct models created after some time to attempt to decide the defenselessness of members to hypnosis.

A portion of the more established profundity scales attempted to construe which level of a daze the member was in through the discernible signs that were accessible. These would incorporate things, for example, the unconstrained amnesia.

A portion of the more present-day scales works to quantify the level of self-assessed or watched responsiveness to the particular recommendation tests that are given, for example, the immediate proposals of unbending arm nature.

As per the examination that has been finished by Deirdre Barrett, there are two kinds of considered profoundly vulnerable subjects that are to the impacts of subliminal therapy.

These two gatherings incorporate dissociates and fantasizers.

The fantasizers will score high on the assimilation scales, will have the option to effortlessly shut out the boosts of this present reality without the utilization of hypnosis, invest a great deal of their energy wandering off in fantasy land, had fanciful companions when they were a youngster, and experienced childhood in a situation where nonexistent play was energized.

Chapter 1

Types of Hypnosis

There are a few innovative methods that hypnosis can be delivered.

1. Guided hypnosis: This type of hypnosis includes using music and recorded instructions to produce a hypnotic state.

2. Hypnotherapy: Hypnotherapy is the type in which hypnosis in psychotherapy is used and is practiced by licensed physicians and psychologists to treat conditions including depression, anxiety, post-traumatic stress disorder (PTSD), and eating disorders.

3. Self-hypnosis: Self-hypnosis is a procedure that takes place when a person hypnotizes itself. It is often used as a self-help technique for managing pain or monitoring stress.

Uses of Hypnosis

Why could an individual decide to try hypnosis? In some cases, to help deal with severe pain or relieve pain and anxiety resulting from medical processes such as surgery or childbirth, people may seek hypnosis.

The following are just a few of the hypnosis applications that have been shown through research:

- Alleviation of irritable bowel syndrome (IBS) related symptoms
- Pain management during dental operations
- Elimination or reduction, including warts and psoriasis, of skin conditions
- Management of certain ADHD symptoms
- Treatment of conditions of chronic pain like rheumatoid arthritis

- Treatment and pain deterioration during childbirth
- Reduction in symptoms of dementia
- Reduction in nausea and vomiting in patients with cancer who undergo chemotherapy

Applications of Hypnosis

The methods used to trigger hypnosis share similar elements. The most significant consideration is that the person (the subject) to be hypnotized is willing and supportive and that he or she trusts the hypnotizer.

To relax in comfort and replace their attentions on some object, subjects are invited. The hypnotist, usually in a low, calm voice, continues to suggest that the relaxation of the subject will boost and that his or her eyes will eventually get tired.

The subject's eyes soon show signs of slowing down, and the hypnotist indicates that they will close. The subject enables his eyes to close and then shows signs of deep relaxation, such as deep breathing and limpness. He has reached the hypnotic state of a haze.

Suppose a person assumes that he may be hypnotized, that the hypnotist is professional and trustworthy, and that the activity is secure, acceptable, and compliant with the subject's desires.

In that case, a person may be more receptive to hypnosis. Induction is, therefore, usually followed by the development of an acceptable partnership between the participant and the hypnotist.

Ordinary hypnosis inductions start with the hypnotist's simple, non-controversial recommendations that all subjects will almost inevitably accept.

At this point, neither the subject nor the hypnotist can easily say if the subject's conduct represents a hypnotic reaction or simple cooperation.

Then, gradually, instructions are offered that require increasing deviation of the individual's perception or memory, e.g., that opening their eyes is hard or impossible for the subject. It can take a long period or just a few seconds for the procedure to take effect.

Based upon the objectives to be fulfilled and the trance's depth, the resultant hypnotic phenomena differ substantially from one subject to another and from one trance to another.

Hypnosis is a hypothesis of degrees, with no fixed constancy, ranging from light to deep trance states. The hypnotist's acceptable ideas will elicit a surprisingly broad variety of neurological, sensory, and motor reactions from profoundly hypnotized individuals.

The subject may be induced to behave as if blind, deaf, paralyzed, hallucinated, amnesic, delusional, or impervious to pain or uncomfortable body postures by accepting and responding to suggestions; besides, the subject may show various behavioral responses that he or she considers to be an appropriate or desirable reaction to the hypnotist's suggested situation.

The posthypnotic suggestion and behavior is one fascinating expression that can be evoked from a subject that has been in a hypnotic trance; that is, the subject's execution, commands, and suggestions given to him while he was in a trance.

The individual will not be aware of the details of his impulse to perform the commanded act, with sufficient amnesia induced during the trance state.

However, a posthypnotic suggestion is not an especially powerful means of controlling behavior than a person's conscious willingness to perform actions.

Many subjects seem incapable of remembering events that occurred while in deep hypnosis. While the subject is in a trance-like state, this "posthypnotic amnesia" can either spontaneously result from deep hypnosis or a hypnotist's recommendation.

Amnesia also includes all or only selected trance-state events or may manifest itself in connection with matters nonrelated to the trance.

By relevant hypnotic suggestions, posthypnotic amnesia may be effectively removed. Medical, dental, psychiatric, and psychological affiliations worldwide have officially endorsed hypnosis as a therapeutic method.

It has been found most helpful in preparing individuals for anesthesia, improving the drug response, and reducing the required dosage. In attempts to stop smoking, hypnosis has often been used and is highly regarded in treating otherwise chronic conditions, including terminal cancer.

It is important to reduce the common fear of dental procedures; in reality, the very people who are most difficult to treat by dentists often respond best to hypnotic suggestions. Hypnosis has been utilized in several contexts in the field of psychosomatic therapy.

Patients have been trained to relieve and to carry out, in the lack of the hypnotist, exercises that have had beneficial impacts on some forms of headaches, high blood pressure, and functional disorders.

Although little training and no specific skills are needed to induce hypnosis, when used in medical treatment, it can be harmful when employed by people who lack the competence and ability to treat such problems without hypnosis.

On the other side, hypnosis has been consistently criticized by numerous medical societies due to the possibility of harmful posthypnotic responses to the treatment. Indeed, many nations have forbidden or restricted commercial or some other public shows of hypnosis in this respect.

Furthermore, many law courts refuse to admit testimony from individuals who have been hypnotized for "recovering" memories because such methods can confuse memories and imaginations.

Impact of Hypnosis

What's the impact of hypnosis? The hypnosis experience can vary dramatically from one person to another.

During the hypnotic state, some hypnotized people report feeling a sense of detachment or extreme relaxation, while others even feel that their actions seem to take place outside of their conscious will. While under hypnosis, other people may remain fully aware and able to carry out conversations.

Researcher Ernest Hilgard's experiments showed how hypnosis could be used to dramatically alter perceptions. The participant's arm was then placed in ice water after instructing a hypnotized person not to feel pain in their arm.

Although non-hypnotized individuals had to expel their arms from the water after a few seconds because of the pain, without experiencing pain, the hypnotized individuals were able to leave their arms in the icy water for several minutes.

Tips

While many individuals believe they cannot be hypnotized, research has shown that many individuals are more hypnotized than they think.

Research suggests that between 10% and 15% of individuals are very responsive to hypnosis.

About 10% of adults are hard or impossible to hypnotize. Kids tend to be more vulnerable to hypnosis. Hypnosis is much more responsive to people who can be readily absorbed in fantasies. It is important to look for a specialist who has credentials and experience in hypnosis as a therapeutic instrument if you are interested in trying hypnotherapy.

It may be useful to look for a psychologist who has been certified by the American Society of Clinical Hypnosis, although many places offer hypnosis training and certification.

Potential Pitfalls

It is common to have misunderstandings about the subject of hypnosis. While amnesia may occur in very rare cases, people generally remember everything that happened while hypnotized.

Hypnosis can, however, have a substantial consequence on memory. Posthypnotic amnesia can go towards a person forgetting some things that happened before or during hypnosis.

This effect is, however, generally restricted, and temporary. While hypnosis can be used to improve memory, the effects of popular media have been dramatically exaggerated.

Research has found that hypnosis does not lead to significant improvement or precision in memory, and hypnosis can lead to false or distorted memories.

Hypnosis does require voluntary involvement on the part of the patient, despite tales about people being hypnotized without their consent.

However, people vary in terms of how hypnotizable and suggestible they are while they are under hypnosis.

Research indicates that, while under hypnosis, highly suggestible individuals are more likely to experience a decreased sense of agency.

While people often feel that without the influence of their will, their activities under hypnosis appear to happen, a hypnotist can't make you perform activities against your wishes.

Although hypnosis can improve performance, it cannot make individuals stronger or more athletic than their current physical abilities.

Risks

A safe, therapeutic, and alternative medicinal therapy is hypnosis performed by a qualified psychiatrist or health care provider.

In individuals with serious mental illness, however, hypnosis may not be acceptable. Hypnosis adverse reactions are uncommon but can include:

- Headaches
- Mental fogginess
- Dizziness
- Distress or fear
- Creation of fake memories

Be alert as hypnosis is suggested as a practice from earlier in life to work during traumatic events. This procedure can evoke intense feelings that can attempt to construct false memories.

History of Hypnosis

The usage of hypnotic-like trance states goes back thousands of years, but through the practice of a psychiatrist called Franz Mesmer, hypnosis started to emerge throughout the late 18th century.

In the late 19th-century, hypnotism became more significant in psychiatry and was utilized by Jean-Martin Charcot to cure women suffering from hysteria.

More recently, to clarify just how hypnosis works, there have been a variety of various hypotheses.

Hilgard's neo-dissociation hypothesis of hypnosis is one of the best-known hypotheses.

According to Hilgard, people in a hypnotic condition undergo a fragmented consciousness in which there are two separate sources of thought.

Although one stream of consciousness reacts to the hypnotist's recommendations, another dissociated stream processes knowledge outside of the hypnotized person's conscious control.

The Ethics of Hypnosis

Hypnotized individuals still have free will, and while they are more open to the recommendation, they will not behave in ways they would usually find morally repugnant.

However, several ethical questions about its use are raised by the nature of hypnosis and how it affects the subconscious.

Are there individuals that can't be hypnotized? It is thought that about 25 percent of the population is not hypnotizable at all.

These people tend to be highly cautious of hypnosis's advantages and unlikely to participate in it willingly.

Can you, and should you, hypnotize yourself? It is possible to do self-hypnosis. While it may be considered cheating or immoral by some, it is a safe way to establish control and start changing unwanted or damaging behaviors.

All it takes for a person to grasp the tools and techniques they must plant healthy hypnotic recommendations in their mind is a quiet place, an open attitude, and practice.

Conditions for Hypnosis to Work Out

How many occasions do you just try to meet your health objectives to have them counteracted with excuses?

It might be that you always find it difficult to wake up in the morning or just postpone doing the routine you choose every day. Even

if you are motivated by coaches, your mindset may only take small steps to change permanently.

Your habits do not come from the subconscious but your conscious mind. Hypnotherapy can be a helpful way of producing changes in the subconscious.

Working with the Subconscious

When it comes to exercise every day, how does hypnotherapy work? The fact that you are unmotivated does not function with hypnotherapy.

While the rational mind is responsible for willpower and thought, 90% of what occurs to us during the day is the subconscious mind's duty.

The subconscious mind acts with illogical cycles of answers and attitudes. While a coach can speak to our conscious mind, the way to circumvent the conscious mind and connect directly to the subconscious is hypnosis.

Changing Behavioral Models

We don't want to work out or make reasons sometimes because fundamental habits deter us from the accomplishment we are aiming for.

Hypnosis instills healthy habits and patterns that make you feel inspired and enthusiastic about going to or working out at the gym quickly.

"Hypnosis will view working out as something exciting to your subconscious rather than something you" must do."

So, through intervention, inspiration would automatically emerge, and you will be the person who cannot wait to hit the gym.

In Hypnosis, You Have the Power

Many people believe that hypnosis is something in which they are beyond any influence and perform everything that they are instructed to do by the hypnotist. This is far from what hypnotherapy is about.

A condition of intense relaxation in hypnosis is mixed with feedback and friendly encouragement in which you are the one directing the process.

In hypnosis, while you are calm, you will enter the secret areas of the conscious mind that block you. We will help you modify the trends that are targeted.

You will have full control of what is happening during the session, and at any point, you can stop the process.

Permanent Results

In all areas of life, including the way you look, regular hypnotherapy can yield permanent results.

Techniques such as visualization and relaxation techniques can help you better care for yourself during hypnotherapy and be more alert to what is going on within your subconscious.

Fitness and exercise will no longer feel like a waste of time before you know it, but something comes to you naturally without stress.

A good workout has many advantages. It can promote better sleep, increase energy, and help you fight illnesses and depression. It can also help you manage stress and produce feel-good hormones called endorphins.

Chapter 2

Benefits of Hypnosis

Hypnosis has become useful when people are surrounded by too much tension in their jobs, and their daily lives are in a rat race. In reality, many people are searching for alternative ways to de-stress and eliminate the many negatives in their lives.

Aside from these stressors in life, several factors prevent a person from being what he wants to be and allowing him to achieve his goals.

Among these are anxiety and anxieties and negative feelings that have been hidden deep inside the subconscious.

One of the methods most people have used these days is hypnosis, and, in reality, it has also been commonly used in the medical industry as a treatment for psychotherapy.

If you're interested in learning more about hypnosis, here are some of the top advantages of hypnosis.

1. Help with phobias and fears. Hypnotherapy has also been effective in resolving deep-rooted fears and phobias that are impossible to conquer consciously. If you don't want to be forced to confront your fears, then hypnosis can be your way to beat it.

2. It helps you to regulate your weight. If you find it very difficult to control your diet and weight, and you lack the motivation to do so, you can find hypnosis as a helpful solution to helping you maintain your weight loss issues.

Most of the time, weight loss attempts fail due to a lack of motivation or control over their emotions.

If you want to support yourself when it comes to losing weight or trying to keep fit, you can also take advantage of the benefits of hypnosis in this field.

3. Overcoming dependency. Another essential application and advantage of hypnosis are helping you conquer addiction and other bad behaviors that are difficult to control consciously.

Alcoholic or opioid abuse are the two most common things that are impossible to manage actively. If you think you're having trouble controlling your addictions, hypnosis will help make the process smoother.

4. Getting rid of the habit of smoking. Yeah, stopping smoking can be very difficult, especially if you've been in the practice for a long time, especially if you're a chain smoker.

If you desire to seek help from your subconscious to reduce the temptations of cigarette lighting, hypnosis can be helpful.

5. Enhancing memory recollection. Memory retrieval is another of the many applications and advantages of hypnosis. This way is also a good use of hypnosis in the courts and in items that require some recall.

Apart from all these applications and advantages of hypnosis, you can also render hypnosis a good tool to boost your ability to manipulate and convince people.

Of course, it is vital that you positively use hypnosis and not hurt anyone. You can also find this useful and helpful, particularly if you're in the sales industry.

Things You Should Know About Hypnosis

Are you considering hypnosis to help you fight a specific life? Good for you, man! Hypnosis is an effective technique to help people solve the issues in their lives.

It is successful over and over in studies and has been endorsed by the American Medical Association, the American Psychiatric Association, and the American Psychological Association for decades. However, there are some things you need to know about hypnosis before you plunge into the process.

Understanding these items ahead of time will help you make the most of whatever work you can do with hypnosis.

1) Hypnosis is a condition of focus and relaxation. Many people have seen hypnosis used in several stage shows, and as a result, they have a somewhat warped understanding of what it is.

It's always believed that a hypnotist will manipulate you or make you do dumb or humiliating stuff, but that's simply not true.

An individual undergoing hypnosis is still in charge and will not do something morally or ethically unacceptable to them.

Hypnosis is a state of absorption, focus, and concentration that makes it easier for us to consider and act on selective, appropriate ideas and suggestions.

(2) You will be able to undergo hypnosis if you want to. Since hypnosis is a state of focus and concentration, if you can do a relatively good job of focusing, you will experience a state of hypnosis.

There appear to be several "hypnotizables," with certain people able to go deeply into hypnotic states and show predictable hypnotic phenomena, and others who have a hard time doing so.

People in the latter group seem to be extremely critical thinkers, but they may also undergo the condition of hypnosis.

People of this bent are typically very good at concentration, so with a specialist used to dealing with a wide variety of individuals, even highly analytical, logical thinkers will undergo hypnosis.

(3) Many people undergo hypnotic environments every day. If you understand the concept of hypnosis as mentioned above, it should be noted that most people experience hypnosis very frequently, maybe even several times a day, and they do!

Any examples: a child who gets so focused on his game system that he doesn't hear his mom calling him for dinner.

Or the partner who is so interested in her computer work that an hour passes, and she feels it's only been 15 minutes.

Or maybe you, when you made the usual drive home from work, and when you pulled into the driveway, couldn't remember the specifics of the drive (this is called "highway hypnosis").

The hypnotist can simply make the process clear and guided for the intent of the improvement that you are seeking.

(4) You can recall what's going on in your hypnosis session. Many people are afraid that they will be in some altered state of consciousness that will not allow them to recognize what's going on during hypnosis, but that's not true.

You will recall, be conscious, and be in charge of the entire process.

(5) Hypnosis is not a magic bullet. Hypnosis is a fantastic way to overcome anxiety, panic, fears, phobias, frustration, depression, or help people lose weight, handle stress better, or develop self-esteem and trust.

But you need to be an enthusiastic and willing participant!

There are several problems where hypnosis is more of an addition to other work that a person does-such as weight loss, so hypnosis would be more effective if you already have a diet and exercise plan in place.

It also requires good communication between you and the professional with whom you work, so be ready to share with him or her what your issues are, what your ambitions are, and any questions you might have along the way.

Treatment of Stress with Self-hypnosis

Why does anyone want to practice self-hypnosis and learn how to do that? One explanation for this is helping to minimize pain.

Getting pain in one's life can be consuming even though it's not persistent. Pain can hurt as well as trigger stress. The problem even takes away the quality of life of a person, whether it's a daily event or every few months, which needs to be monitored.

Different people have different causes for their suffering from a disease to injury. It can be handled with medication occasionally.

However, this drug can't work for everybody, or you may prefer to treat the pain without medication. One way to do this is to increase the popularity of self-hypnosis. This technique is thought to put a stop to the discomfort.

Well, if you haven't seen a doctor for the pain, it may be a good idea to get started. This way is to make sure there's nothing serious about the problem that the doctor wants to handle.

It's also going to help you know the root of the pain. Now, you can focus on that painful spot.

The use of self-hypnosis only treats pain, not the real cause.

You will still feel better and struggle less. It may also be used by others to work with their medications.

Self-hypnosis also works instantly, and an important note of pain relief can be seen when used regularly.

It is recommended that this procedure be implemented at the beginning of each day. There are ways to learn about self-hypnosis from books to experts. Knowing how to do self-hypnosis correctly ensures that there is a greater chance of it working.

When someone knows the process and tries it over and over again, it's going to be simpler. It's all down to what you think is going to work for you. You can try self-hypnosis, whether you like it or not.

Some individuals pursue self-hypnosis and give it a shot, but find it doesn't work for them.

They're choosing to try something else. Others take self-hypnosis to help relieve pain. They discover that they like it, and it works for them.

They learned the right technique, and they were able to bring it into their everyday routine. Many feel it won't hurt to try self-hypnosis, particularly if they're in such pain, they think they don't have a choice, and nothing else helps.

Also, self-hypnosis helps relieve stress and is one of the techniques used to relieve stress at home and in the corporate world.

Weight Loss through Hypnosis and Other Techniques

Obesity is not just the gathering of the abundance of muscle versus fat. Stoutness is an interminable (long-term) illness with genuine confusion that is exceptionally hard to treat.

Accordingly, it requires long-haul treatment to get more fit and keep it off. There is no medium-term arrangement. Powerful, changeless weight reduction takes some time.

The fundamental factors in getting more fit and keeping it off are inspiration, legitimate eating, practice propensities, and energy about better wellbeing.

Getting in shape will enable you to feel much improved. It likewise will improve your wellbeing.

Heftiness is the subsequent driving reason for preventable deaths in the United States driven by tobacco. A long way from the broadly referenced techniques used to get more fit lies other unmentioned goliaths.

Hypnosis and Weight Loss

Hypnosis is an instrument a few specialists use to enable people to arrive at a condition of complete unwinding.

During a session, professionals accept that the cognizant and oblivious personality can concentrate and focus on verbal reiteration and mental symbolism.

The brain, accordingly, ends up open to recommendation and open to change concerning practices, feelings, and propensities.

Types of this elective treatment have been utilized since the 1700s to help individuals with anything from bed-wetting to nail gnawing to smoking.

Research on hypnosis has likewise demonstrated some guarantee for treating corpulence, as we will investigate in this piece. It is not about another person controlling your psyche and causing you to accomplish interesting things while you are oblivious.

You do not lose control of your psyche during hypnosis. You are likewise not oblivious when you experience trance—it is progressively similar to an underground government of unwinding.

Being in that state makes you progressively powerless to change, and that is the reason trance for weight reduction might be compelling.

Early examinations from the 90s found that individuals who utilized hypnosis lost more than twice as much weight as the individuals who consumed fewer calories without subjective treatment.

A recent report worked with 60 fat women and found that the individuals who rehearsed Hypno-behavioral treatment shed pounds and improved their dietary patterns and self-perception.

Furthermore, a little 2017 investigation worked with eight fat grown-ups and three youngsters, every one of whom effectively shed pounds, with one, in any event, keeping away from the medical procedure because of the treatment benefits.

The perfect competitor is any individual who experiences difficulty adhering to a sound eating regimen and exercise program since they cannot shake their negative propensities.

Here is a portion of the means you can pursue:

Stage 1

Discover a time in your day where you will not be diverted by outside variables. Attempt to put aside in any event 30 minutes where you can inundate yourself in a stupor. It is imperative to center during this whole timeframe.

Stage 2

Set weight reduction objectives for yourself. Go for an accurate measure of weight you need to lose and explicit time you need to lose it

Stage 3

Picture yourself as the size you need to be. Envision what your body will resemble once you accomplish your optimal weight. Additionally, consider how others will respond and what they will say.

Stage 4

Close your eyes and loosen up your body until it is limp.

Stage 5

Envision your optimal self in a dazed state. Consider how you will see the world, how others will see you, and how great it will feel to be solid and fit as a fiddle. Take a gander at your body in its slender, trim state.

Stage 6

Return to your present state gradually. Be certain you bring the sentiments of the inward experience back with you.

Doing this day by day will prepare your psyche to feel how great it will be to lose weight. You will progressively make the conduct adjustments important to get thinner.

You do not need to be enchanted to gain proficiency with a portion of the precious exercises that mesmerizing needs to instruct about weight reduction.

Subliminal specialists trust you have all that you have to succeed. You do not generally require another accident diet or the most recent hunger suppressant.

Thinning is tied in with confiding in your intrinsic capacities, as you do when you ride a bike; it was hard from the outset yet as you continued, everything else fell set up consequently.

Individuals will, in general, accomplish what they want to accomplish. That even applies to mesmerizing.

A smart thought is to have a perpetual wellspring of creative mind for what might be on the horizon.

Envisioning a day of good dieting encourages you to imagine the fundamental strides to turning into that sound eater. If you experience difficulty envisioning this, locate an old photo of yourself at an agreeable weight and recollect what you were doing another way at that point; envision restoring those schedules. Consider what you are doing diverse right now.

Quietly rehashing a positive affirmation 15 to 20 minutes every day can change your eating, particularly when joined with moderate, regular breaths, the foundation of any social change program.

One entrancing session cannot get down to the business of your eating routine, careful discipline brings about promising results. In case of a backslide, celebrate.

Try not to put yourself down more than you have as of now. Keep in mind, a collection of stress may have driven you to the way you are right now. You would prefer not to sink yourself more profound than you are as of now.

Spellbinding perspectives a backslide as a chance, not a crime.

If you can gain from a genuine or envision backslide - why it occurred, how to deal with it unexpectedly - you will be better arranged forever's unavoidable enticements. Make a point to have some good times while sending your nourishment yearnings away.

Once more, hypnosis is all right for a great many people. Unfriendly responses are uncommon. Potential dangers include hallucinations, nervousness, laziness, unsteadiness, and migraines.

Individuals who experience mental trips or daydreams ought to address their primary care physician before difficult hypnotherapy. Additionally, entrancing ought not to be performed on a person affected by medications or liquor.

It may not be fruitful.

If you attempt it exclusively with a doctor, your specialist will probably start your session by clarifying how mesmerizing functions.

They will at that point go over your objectives. From that point, your specialist may start talking in an alleviating, delicate voice to enable you to unwind and to set up a sentiment of wellbeing.

When you have arrived at a progressively open perspective, your advisor may propose approaches to enable you to change you are eating or exercise propensities or different approaches to arrive at your weight reduction objectives.

Certain words or reiteration of specific expressions may help with this stage. Your specialist may likewise enable you to imagine yourself arriving at objectives through sharing striking mental symbolism.

To close the session, your advisor will help take you out of entrancing and back to your beginning state.

The length of the entrancing session and the number of all-out sessions you may need will rely upon your objectives. A few people may get results in as few as one to three sessions.

Chapter 3

Techniques to reach your ideal weight

Getting absorbed into your ideas and thoughts is that gentle trip to the middle of yourself self-known as "entering a trance."

The natural methods of self-hypnosis contain entering trance, broadening the trance, together with this trance, provide suggestions and messages into this mind-body, and coming from the trance.

Moving into Trance

Whenever you're employing the trancework about the sound, it will become your guide when you enter a trance.

I'll use a trance induction procedure; you will discover focusing and relaxing. You've likely noticed the swinging view approach in films.

However, there are lots of unique methods to focus your focus on entering the trance.

You may stare at a place on the wall, then use a breathing procedure, or use innovative body comfort. You may hear various induction approaches on the trancework sound.

They're only the clues or the signs which you're committing to saying, "I'm entering trance" or even" I will perform my negativity today."

Moving into trance may also be considered as "permitting yourself to daydream... intentionally".

You're letting yourself become consumed into your ideas, really consumed, and letting yourself pretend or imagine what you want as real and achieved. There's no "going under." Instead, there's a beautiful experience of moving inside.

Deepening the Trance

Deepening your trance makes it possible to become more absorbed into your mind, thoughts, and expertise. It can be done with innovative comfort, heading "deeper and deeper inside."

With scenes or images, or only by simply counting a few chains.

We love to indicate as you listen to the counting down to zero, then you produce a vertical vision that's connected with moving deeper, including a path resulting in a hill or to a lush green valley.

Since you hear me, you can envision or imagine going deeper into a spectacle or location that's even more comfortable and enjoyable to you. That is what we mean by "deepening the trance."

Talking into the Mind of Your Own Body with Messages and Tips

Throughout the trancework, you may listen to your voice talking to 2 components of your mind. 1 portion of your brain is the conscious mind thoughts.

That's the part of you who is great at telling the time, making change, understanding how to write and read. It's "thinking thoughts."

Through the trancework, your believing thoughts will keep on performing their regular activity of getting ideas.

So, that you do not need to be worried about clearing your head, or draining your head, or placing your mind entirely at peace? Just see your thoughts will last "believing," and your task is to disconnect or unplug only enough, so you don't need to respond to those notions. You permit them to flow by.

If your "to-do" list keeps popping up, for example, simply let it flow by instead of life on it. Another portion of the mind I'll be talking to you about is that we predict your subconscious thoughts "sub" since it's under your belief degree of consciousness.

It's that the "mind of the physique." Your subconscious mind has the knowledge to handle your body's trillions of cells, your body chemistry, and all of the body's acts of breathing, digestion, and the nervous system, the endocrine system, and also the immune system.

The mind-body has a massive quantity of wisdom. Also, in performing your hypnosis, you're amassing and obtaining additional knowledge the thoughts of your own body will act upon, consistent with your motivation, your own beliefs, along with your expectations, and assisting you with your weight reduction.

You have the chance to correct and tailor the phrases being discussed, or the graphics described to best match you.

This tailoring procedure is essential. It must fit you personally since it's your self-hypnosis, and all of the hypnosis is self-hypnosis.

As we have mentioned, hypnosis isn't something to you. It is something that you are being advised to encounter, and since you encounter it, you're learning it. Repeating and rehearsal produce strong knowledge and ability inside you.

Perhaps you will call it unconscious understanding as your subconscious mind might take it out to you without you needing to think of it.

So, the ideas which might have been bothering you about your weight loss, or your inability to shed weight, are presently being shifted into something which supports your ideal body.

Along with your mind-body memorizing the encounter so it may refer to this adventure rather than the undesirable outcomes of the past.

For example, if you believe That You're a more "yo-yo" dieter since you have always recovered the weight you've lost. You might use your trancework to indicate:

"Every single day I'm losing weight, along with my entire body, remembers the way to make this a lasting ability. I'm achieving my ideal weight".

Subconscious comprehension or even the mind-body wisdom that's learned from the trancework is much like choosing to ride a bike or drive a vehicle.

When you're learning, there appeared to be lots of things to look closely at precisely the same time.

However, quite fast you're hard-won on this understanding so that you will be able to drive. And you don't even need to inform your toes precisely what to do.

Coming from Trance

At the close of the trancework sessions, you may hear me talking about allowing your body to wake up with a sense of refreshment and well-being.

Also bringing this refreshment with you to the surface of the mind, so you come from trance feeling renewed and awake. Or, when performing your hypnosis at nighttime, you might drift into a deep, relaxed sleep.

Once you're alert, it's crucial to debrief.

Here is the opportunity to create a note or two on your ideas or thoughts that came to mind that will be handy to you.

Frequently during childbirth, not just are you providing messages into your own body, but also your body is speaking to you personally, and you'll be listening to the thoughts of your body.

Your body can reveal quite beneficial info, and you might choose to write it all down. For instance, let's suppose you have a specific food which you just cannot resist, a meal such as French Fries, which was the "downfall" of dieting.

Throughout the trancework, you might find an insight (something you noticed when you listened to the brain of your own body) that lets you know French Fries became an obstruction or a "relaxation" for you mentally.

That insight today permits you to pick what you would like rather than only execute the prior pattern, which has been established possibly decades ago and created from a subjective experience that's long ago and no more legitimate in your lifetime.

Jennifer was meticulous and hardworking in each area of her life, along with virtually every aspect of her burden loss program. She exercised daily, ate plenty of produce, drank lots of water, loved grains, as well as purchased organic material.

She made quite wise decisions for wellness but stayed twenty pounds within her ideal weight.

As she sat in our workplace, she told her insatiable appetite for ice cream (natural though it had been) every evening and in each social opportunity that presented itself.

Throughout her trance work, we inquired if there had been a component of her, why she appeared to crave ice cream.

She had been quiet for many moments, then reiterated the long-ago words of her adoring grandfather: "Jenny, beloved, ice cream would be the ideal reward for hard labor, so she consumes while it continues. "After she discovered the origin of her ice hockey lotion urge, she managed to appreciate it but not consume it often.

What was the Experience Like for You?

Now that you've had experience using self-hypnosis, what did you encounter? Are you currently "hypnotized"?

Can you go to a hypnotic trance? Nearly all people that are new to hypnosis will wonder whether they experienced it. You might feel precisely the same.

If you were anticipating a profoundly changed state of awareness, then you've found that there is no "going under" without a loss of awareness.

You know where you were, what you're doing, if not all the moment. We hear the same testimony whenever people have finished their initial encounter with self-hypnosis: "This was wonderful (or amazing, or exceptional, or impressive)."

When I'm asked what I encounter when in a trance, a good illustration from my school years comes into mind, I had been looking outside the window during a lecture.

I wouldn't understand what the professor was lecturing, but I might listen to his voice. However, I didn't have any idea what he had been saying through those minutes.

Being trance is very similar to being in a daydream country.

The significant difference between a trance and a daydream is that a trance is a deliberate kind of daydream wherein you're consumed in thoughts that you need your mind-body to discuss.

When in mind, you experience an aim to supply your mind-body with suggestions or ideas about what you would like it to do to you personally.

We're always thrilled to hear folks say following their very first trance encounter, "I enjoyed it. I didn't want it to end." We understand that when a seasoned trance is found, they could take action.

Hypnotic Phenomena

Trance is a delicate experience. You can examine the subtleties of what you believed, what you discovered, not discovering, and what you've experienced.

Some could feel heavy, their legs and arms could be immovable, or they might feel mild, weightless, or even drifting. Some may feel cool or warm or be absorbed in the emotional imagery they feel like they are within their vision.

Regions of the human body may appear to vanish so wholly they aren't even detected. It's also common to experience some time. One minute might look like ten minutes, or ten minutes might seem like just one. All these are ordinary experiences we predict "hypnotic phenomena."

If you're conversant with daydreaming, you know that many of what's known as hypnotic phenomena can also be common waking-state phenomena.

How frequently have you ever "awakened" out of a daydream, or even been roused in an intriguing book or film, to discover that a surprising quantity of time has elapsed?

The available array of happenings with misuse is extensive, such as hypoalgesia (the decrease in pain) and also hypoaesthesia (the removal of annoyance).

When in a trance, a person may imagine a part or all her body is indeed readily numb that she can undergo a surgical procedure using hypnosis as the only anesthetic.

You'll be pleased to know that hypnotic phenomena could be generated, especially helpful for weight reduction. You could have the ability to make, for example, a physical feeling of fullness, or even a craving for food that is wholesome.

You could have the ability to make a feeling of improved taste or odor. You might even have the ability to overlook foods that aren't consistent with your weight reduction objectives. You might even be surprised to feel a craving for the exercise.

Bear in mind the ability of self-hypnosis. It is possible to select what you would like to convey for your mind-body.

It is possible to choose what you need your mind-body to perform for you. It's your option, your ideal weight.

Chapter 4

Hypnosis Portion Control Session

Habits control our lives and not only form our present life, but also define the shape of our future.

Portion management is known to be one of the main factors that people accumulate weight, and while for others, that does not make logical sense, it is something that will greatly affect the path to losing weight.

You want to be in charge of your mind through hypnotherapy, which will help you to better charge the behaviors and patterns you have. There are many explanations for why individuals overeat.

Many cannot even claim that individuals make a choice to do so, which suggests why unmindful feeding is often considered.

Is Management Of Portions Hard To Maintain?

Yeah, if you don't know what you place in your mouth. If you have ever heard the phrase, "Anything too much isn't good for you," you'll realize it's the reality.

You should question yourself, after consuming something tiny or a big meal, "Did that meal make me feel good?" Does it support my body, and would it serve me in every conceivable way other than making sure I'm full?

Buffet meals have been a regular practice at restaurants. Why else do individuals have the urge to feed as much as they do?

Many clinicians will highlight the point that their patients and individuals in general, have psychological challenges that contribute to unhealthy behaviors, such as overeating, sometimes forgetting or resolving mental trauma, emotions, and unfinished concerns.

It doesn't matter what the motivations might be, overeating is not deemed safe, and it may impact the body adversely, aside from allowing your body to add weight.

It may also lead to health conditions that can be recognized with signs such as acid reflux, frequently feeling uncomfortably loaded, water accumulation, and abdominal area visceral fat relatively high.

Needless to mention, behaviors are in charge of our lifestyles, and we are more likely than we would like to confess to overeat. The U.S. is the prime illustration of a nation that has built a community of normalizing portions that are too big to be eaten by an individual.

It is the standard, though, which has led to over half of the inhabitants suffering either from obesity or becoming overweight. What individuals ought to comprehend is that obesity is not deemed a form of a body.

It is deemed a major health concern that may cause many other health conditions.

Heart disease, diabetes, elevated blood pressure, stroke, cancer, gallbladder disorder, gallstones, gout, osteoarthritis, and respiratory complications, including sleep apnea and asthma, are among these health problems.

The explanation that portion management is deemed complicated is that we consume for all the wrong reasons.

Society is vulnerable to gravitating to diets containing an unbalanced amount of sugar, salt, fatty fats, and calorie content. These goods are therefore advertised as more enticing and are marketed while our eyes are feasting similarly.

Individuals are still accustomed to overeating and have grown to accept it as a terrible behavior that they can not manage to get rid of.

People also assume that they can't afford to waste food or feel obligated to finish everything they have on their table. Other than that, it has been treated as natural to overeat.

Seeing that individuals are more bored, unhappy, or mentally distressed than ever before, it still seems like the safest choice to consume anything they might find or go for the wrong alternative.

Portion management, since it may identify us from being safe or bad, plays a very significant role in our well-being.

It affects the relation of our bodies to how much we weigh and lets us hang on to extra weight. If you practice a sort of 'balanced' diet and a fair exercise schedule, often go back to review if you consume sufficient or too much and if you are conscious of your eating habits.

Not only does managing your portions allow for a thinner body, but it also supplies you with more resources and improves your metabolism.

The more calories you give your body, the longer it may work to absorb it, which is why, after overeating, you will feel slow and lazy.

It requires a lot of work to meet increased food intake requirements and may cause the metabolism to decelerate as a way of protecting itself against damage.

Hypnosis encourages you to rediscover harmony with your food patterns, helping you to be in sync with your priorities and concentrate on them. In this way, together with your self-confidence and development, you can also recover your self-worth that might have been lost.

By submitting to hypnosis, you will do all of this and more.

Hypnosis is often known to be much more successful for weight reduction and some form of mind-body interaction, pushing that a stage further, when it has been found to have an efficacy rate of up to 93 percent relative to all forms of treatment (Meridian Peak Hypnosis, n.d.).

The numbers alone could make everyone want to pursue hypnosis that is combined with food regulation.

While several diet and exercise plans are advertised online, some of them are also made accessible free of charge; the mind begins with the best path to lose weight.

Hypnosis is a method of sustainable weight reduction that allows us access to our unconscious mind, removes all hurdles, and replaces them with concepts that are more valuable than any kind of knowledge.

Hypnosis often helps one to delve deep within our brains, just as though we were testing the archives on our devices, and to get rid of any unpleasant memories in the creation of new behaviors that we may have.

How To Overcome Difficulties With Portion Size And Overeating

Food is essential for life, so where would the need for food get to a stage where overeating and overindulging results? When should you evaluate yourself, pause for a moment and refrain from eating?

It is regarded likewise by every person who has an unhealthy interaction with food. It also acts as a source of comfort and protection that helps us to reassure ourselves that eating food carelessly and without thought is appropriate.

Needless to mention, you don't have a particularly good experience with food unless you are educated in food or educate yourself in the principle of thinking for your well-being.

If you have identified the desire to develop a healthier food partnership, and you want to find out more about weight loss hypnosis and knock your poor behaviors, you need to determine the root trigger leading to your dilemma.

Since eating is a means of temporary stress relief and diverts us from experiencing emotions such as stress, depression, anxiety, and frustration, at least at some stage in our lifetime, it is something we seem to gravitate towards.

Since advertisement firms are specialists in introducing faulty foods to us that might look desirable or are wrapped in relatively "dietary-friendly" material, we have accepted the idea that fake food consumption or whatever advertisement implies to us is good.

We also told ourselves similarly that eating fast food serves as a reward for everything we do well.

For starters, it is incorrect to convince yourself that after six weekdays of clean eating, you can eat anything you want on Sunday.

By consuming a safe, nutritious meal, we should not think like we are starving ourselves.

When we follow a healthier lifestyle, it can become part of the routine. The first move to effectively utilizing hypnosis for weight reduction is to recognize the causes that you are unable to accomplish whatever it is you desire.

You must understand how to resolve your food problem while doing self-hypnosis to transform it into something beneficial, such as encouragement not to feel as frail or miserable as you do at your present weight or physical condition.

You should understand the explanation why your target feels so out of sight before you proceed with your practice, and also what it is that keeps you back from meeting it. A professional would usually ask you a series of questions relating to weight management, plus questions regarding your food and workout patterns, during a clinical hypnotherapy session.

You should easily go over your everyday life and routines as you are working out the counseling session on your own. Often, knowing that you need to change, assists in writing down both good and harmful behaviors.

During the session, you need to set out all the details next to you and reflect on what you'd like to change.

Setting down your plans would also allow you to build a better image of where you intend to go. Please remember that self-hypnosis is completely up to you because, over the 21 days, you have to concentrate and remain focused.

Most people will hit this time and set a benchmark for themselves without trying to create a promise that is too high.

It's crucial, to be frank about unhealthy behavior with yourself because you have to rectify your food problem, which may be everything from binge feeding, emotional eating, overeating, or manipulating yourself to feel that you need additional food or more often seen as an excuse, convincing yourself that on Monday you're going to start a plan.

Obtaining the appropriate details about yourself and your behaviors can help to uncover and reflect on what you need to fix.

Participating in hypnotherapy, you would be able to strengthen your confidence by constructive feedback to help you feel inspired, reboot your inner voice, encouraging you to sustain an optimistic and safe attitude, imagine yourself meeting your objectives of weight reduction, recognize implicit habits that lead to your present unhealthy weight, and get hold of any apprehension you might have in. You certainly didn't realize you could operate in danger of accomplishing your objectives.

It seems ridiculous, but it may also be stressful to adjust yourself or the way you work.

Individuals also don't fulfill their ambitions, and they are scared to abandon their comfort bubble. Because, without becoming miserable in life, we will not prosper or grow, it is essential to resolve such fears.

Hypnosis can tackle your routines and encourage you to eliminate them from your subconscious mind. It will enable you to establish new and permanent strategies for coping.

With hypnosis, for instance, you may imagine yourself reacting to a difficult interaction or circumstance and chose how you want to behave safely.

To help you make healthier decisions and shape lasting eating patterns, you can even picture yourself eating well during the exercise.

It's easy to keep to their routine form of eating for those who don't compete for portion and craving regulation.

Hypnosis is perhaps the greatest form of self-development, relative to someone who is compulsive and feeds depending on their emotions.

It operates by managing perceptions and patterns that have undoubtedly contributed to your diet pitfalls and dysfunctional relationships.

You are advised during the hypnosis process to determine a way to dispatch the sugar cravings and eradicate unhealthy behavior around portion control.

This allows you to imagine yourself getting a far better food experience, and will set you up for success.

For hypnosis, solely concentrating on actively dropping weight sounds stupid. There are so many more variables involved that you should correct the characteristics of what induces weight gain.

A process that will put you on the road to living your better life is reducing weight and reaching every health-related target.

How To Consume The Appropriate Quantity Of Food

You ought to work on consuming the right kinds of food to restore reasonable portion sizes and consume the optimal quantity of food.

You will only be able to sustain a healthy diet then. Before you proceed with hypnosis, it is often beneficial to perform a little study, particularly if you aim to learn how to limit your food portions and adhere to it.

Although you realize why you should and why consuming so much food adds to the excessive accumulation of fat that is accumulated in the body, many individuals will overeat anyway.

It's important to note that you are not meant to live to eat, but instead to feed to live.

You can regulate your food portions after you've developed this principle, and, hopefully, lose some weight.

 If you are doing hypnosis or are currently adopting a diet and you don't lose weight, then your food portions will have to be evaluated.

You will have to adapt to your body to understand whether the kind of food you consume suits your health well.

The consequence of unhealthy eating at meals, maybe the extra weight.

Overeating too often is also the same as consuming a bad diet; it's not beneficial for your physical wellbeing or your path towards weight reduction. Appropriate portion management alone can't help you drop all the weight, but it will offer you more stamina, especially when our body systems are continually straining from full places to function harder.

This involves your appetite, which may allow you to hang on to extra weight if you don't function well, stop your weight reduction efforts entirely, and lead you to feel insecure.

It may be a severe health condition to have a slow metabolism and poor digestion, causing harmful signs such as persistent fatigue, weight gain, stress, vomiting, constipation, and cravings for sweets.

The word "portion management" applies to consume an appropriate quantity of food. If your purpose is weight loss, the amount of what you eat, together with the nature of it, is considered.

Sometimes, out of kindness or just because we can't accept the fact that we have had enough, individuals push themselves to consume the food on their table.

You should start using the following to monitor your portion sizes:

- Feed gradually and be more mindful of what you consume.
- 15 minutes before dining, consume a glass of water. It would load your stomach and, in one sitting, keep you from consuming too much.
- Skip buffets at restaurants or eat 2-for-1 offers. -- Use a smaller tray.
- Take your meal pictures and store them in a database so that you can physically revisit and equate the scale of your meals. It can also assist you to keep on board and strive to progress.

Why Hypnosis Functions For The Management Of Portions

The above strategies for managing your portion sizes during meals may be incorporated, but you also need to try to resolve unhealthy behaviors.

Consuming compulsively is nothing to be proud of, and food must be treated as energy. Improving the nature of the food also assists with the management of portions, which will enable you to make the best choices.

Let's be honest; no one wants to eat a huge broccoli dish.

Focusing on how you feel when consuming tiny or big volumes of food can also help you resolve any mental conflict or need to ingest the correct servings of food.

You will enter a profoundly peaceful state of mind and feel motivated if you continue to overcome your problems with portion management, since you may not feel like you have to resolve your unconsciousness anymore. Now you're going to be in charge.

It is a huge obstacle to conquer portion management, but it is not something that can't be done. In culture nowadays, it is extremely challenging to do.

In the last 50 years, what used to be called acceptable portion sizes have now multiplied.

It has also been normalized because there is a new generation of individuals, and has been one of the key contributions to elevated instances of obesity.

You ought to indulge in mindfulness to overcome whatever dilemma you might have linked to consuming so many calories a day, whether it's overeating or consuming empty calories.

This is something that only you can teach yourself. It is not a talent, but instead an act of stepping back and recognizing what you are doing, even the amount of what you eat, for example.

Hypnosis Session For Portion Management

In this portion control hypnosis session, we will concentrate on six variables to incorporate into your everyday life, which can help you make healthier decisions about dietary choices, and also the amount of food you eat.

Although this hypnosis session's aim is not primarily to lose weight but simply to consume less, knowing how to regulate your calories will boost up your metabolism and make you enjoy a healthier quality of life overall.

The six aspects we will reflect on throughout this session include:

1. Focus on healthy nutrition-You can learn how to adopt a new eating style that focuses on reducing your appetite and accelerating your metabolism.
    This program aims to consume six small meals a day, with a combination of carbs, protein, and vegetables. You will concentrate on making what you feel to be the best day in your head in this session, in which you visualize yourself consuming fewer calories at meals.
2. Focus on shrinking your stomach-For portion management sessions, you can focus on contemplating getting a tiny stomach by incorporating deep breathing into the hypnosis. You can think about yourself as having a tinnier, flatter stomach whenever you breathe in. You would be able to manipulate your mind into believing that you like this picture of yourself, provided that you choose this model over your current appearance.

3. Monitor the cravings, like sweets and fast-food cravings, as well as consuming too much at one go. Concentrate on consuming steadily. By creating a timeline in which you end your snack or dinner, this can be achieved. You do not hurry to feed. You'll be able to alleviate the cravings by concentrating on feeding steadily.

4. Focus on consuming water-Drinking water to load up your stomach can serve a vital role in helping you conquer portion sizes, acting as among the most beneficial strategies to alleviate cravings and over-eating. Since consuming water will also allow you to get rid of disorders like tension, nausea, asthma, intestinal disorders, and depression, it would fit you much better than feeding yourself whole.

5. Focus on greens and the vegetables-The odds are that you eat the wrong kinds of food because you eat so much food. Nobody needs to consume a large portion of vegetables, as I suggested earlier.
That's why it's a particularly smart idea to load your plate with 50% of veggies and leafy greens to make you believe you're already physically consuming enough food. For lunch, you may eat a salad the size of a standard plate, but you can't have a tray of chips the size of a lunch tray. Plus, you won't continue to consume too much food until you integrate healthier eating into your everyday life, and you can learn the importance of it.

6. Concentrate on the sensation of hunger-You must remember hunger throughout your hypnosis session for portion management. If you're not hungry, then you're not going to feed, and if you think like you're not supposed to be hungry since you fed a little earlier, before shifting to food, drink a glass of water. Concentrate on what your body requires when you are hungry, though, and not what is either easy or sounds better than a healthy choice. It is also really useful and

essential to find foods that are safe to add to your everyday diet. It could be the distinction between whether you adhere to a balanced eating schedule or not.

Chapter 5

Mini habits for great results

Occasionally we can feel out of control In regards to eating. We feel pressured to go on fad diets, or even work out extra hard in the gym.

Even though it's extremely important to exercise and watch what you eat, it is equally critical that you build a great relationship with meals. This will determine the level of your life, both at the office and at home.

A healthy relationship with Food requires effort, but working towards feeling more at peace with ingesting is worth it. Here is what you could do to avoid unhealthy habits from ongoing.

Be flexible.

"Our minds like to Consider in Vintage stipulations," states Susan Albers, author of 50 Ways to Soothe Yourself Without Food. "Right vs. Wrong. Fat versus lean.

Perfect versus destroyed." If you slide on a diet, do not let yourself mentally spiral. While this occurs, you'll end up overthinking, overeating, as well as thinking all kinds of negative thoughts and decisions on your own.

Think about being strict with what you consume. Albers advises to occasionally split your diet even only a little bit--as being elastic can alleviate a lot of the stress you might feel.

And, as she notes, "When you notice that nothing awful happens, flexibility will not be intimidating. Perhaps you will like it."

Be attentive.

When would you overeat or eat bad food? Can a particular event or feeling activate your unhealthy eating habits?

Occasionally, by way of instance, we crave particular foods if we are tired at work, and we visit the vending machine to solve the craving.

Be mindful of your hunger triggers and cues when you eventually notice and focus on some unhealthy eating patterns, you're able to effectively purge them.

Be relaxed.

Maintain a comfortable approach when it Comes to meals, not only does that aid with weight care. However, also, it enables you to make progress with your health all around.

Relaxed eating makes it possible to eat till you are nutritionally pleased and helps facilitate emotional eating, therefore look at slowing down through all foods, lunch at your desk.

Inspect different textures, tastes, and elements of your meals, and overall love.

Stop punishing yourself for everything you ate.

It is not serving you personally or your physique! In reality, your entire body reacts to the negative jumble, which generates undesirable stress in the body! Stress is the number one health killer.

Practice mindful eating.

Look at it. Taste it. Smell it. Use your perceptions! Enjoy what's on the plate. This way, your brain will indicate"satiety," and you will be less inclined to overeat.

Relish your food.

Don't cloud your consumption experience With negative ideas such as, "I shouldn't be eating this" or even"I am a loser that I couldn't control what I ate." Your own body will manifest those ideas into physiological stress! Hi, cortisol!!!

Goodbye to optimum digestion! Please, be in peace with your plate.

Stop the vicious cycle of all-or-nothing.

Should you make a poor food choice, attempt To let it all go! Your entire body reacts to everything you do the majority of the time, maybe not occasionally!

The majority of us think, "well, I ate which donut so that I may as well keep moving" this turns into what's called a 'food binge.' Now see that is where the problem appears.

That your body doesn't mind the donut so much, but it is going to begin to mind all of the rest, which you simply fill it with. It just does not understand exactly what to do with it all at one time.

Practice positive affirmations.

Affirmations are a powerful instrument to Reverse negative ideas and reprogram your beliefs, actions, and behavior.

They could alter how you find the planet and most certainly helped me improve my relationship with my physique:

- This plate of food is really great for me.
- My body knows how to utilize this food.
- My cells are all going to be not nourished with this much goodness.

Give up the need to eat and be absolute.

Nobody eats perfectly. Perfect does not exist! Try out a release that wants and remember you're good enough.

Quit comparing!

Your body and nutrient demands are Different from those of your friends, your sister, and your mom! Their relationship with food doesn't have anything to do with you.

They have entirely different and elaborate body mechanics. You can't take their relationship with their meals, my love!

Do not be difficult with meals.

It is important not to allow your Healthful lifestyle to get in the way of your life. (I try really hard for this one!)

If you are outside with family and friends, do not be concerned about the food choices. It is not important.

Just select the finest available for you. Otherwise, you may just complicate your relationship with meals.

If you are reaching for food when you are not hungry afterward, something emotional is happening.

Why are you reaching that Relaxation? Just spot it. If you understand you are not hungry, I urge you to do something else that is pleasurable!

Go for a walk, massage, spa, Paint your nails, be romantic with your spouse, watch your favorite TV series with a cuppa, have a talk for your bestie, or move stalk some wellness sites and write off your fave recipes! Anything!

Hypnosis for Weight Loss: Using Hypnotherapy to Shed Pounds

Close your eyes, breath, unwind. Envision yourself fighting the temptation to enjoy. Envision you never again ache for undesirable nourishments. Envision you never again want to comfort yourself with nourishment.

If the weight loss was that straightforward, you might be thinking. If no one but you could "turn off" your unfortunate yearnings...

That is the possibility of hypnosis for weight loss. Using hypnotherapy, those hoping to lose weight are engaged to refresh the programmed musings that trigger nourishment desires.

Overeating and overindulgence will, in general, be related in our psyches with specific sentiments, connections, and events.

What's more, our minds have persuaded us that in specific circumstances, nourishment fills a basic need – for example utilizing nourishment to comfort pressure.

At last, to accomplish long haul weight reduction, we should get to these oblivious hindrances, evacuate them, and supplant these programmed considerations with increasingly accommodating data.

Hypnotherapy engages us to get to these programmed contemplations, erase the negative affiliations, and create positive affiliations that can assist us with accomplishing long-term weight reduction achievement.

How Food Invades the Mind: Overcoming the Mental Barriers

State Clara begins an eating routine. Also, it's going solid. She's two weeks or three weeks it – has to lose weight, and she feels extraordinary.

However, at that point, something changes. Clara begins a new position. Presently, she thinks that it's increasingly hard to lose. She's overindulging all the more regularly, quit tallying calories, and she's hankering undesirable nourishments.

Her weight loss slows down, and after a short time, she's tumbled off the eating routine. What turned out badly? Clara began so solid, yet couldn't remain on track.

If we investigate this at a more profound level, we may reveal a "habit pattern" that offers a clarification.

Habit patterns structure through reiteration, and after some time, they become oblivious reactions to improvements or conditions. Right now, likely built up a propensity example of stress eating, which kept her from contacting her weight loss goals.

Nourishment had become Clara's oblivious, automatic reaction to stretch. These sorts of propensities for the mind are actually why getting more fit is such a test for a significant number of us.

Somewhere down in our unconscious minds, we've created solid thoughts regarding unfortunate practices.

Actually, after some time, we may have prepared the psyche to accept that these unfortunate practices are basic – that they are important for keeping up our prosperity.

Also, if the mind accepts these practices are fundamental, long-term change is troublesome.

Stress or passionate eating is only one model. There are numerous affiliations that we build up that contrarily sway our relationship to nourishment.

Some regular affiliations that forestall weight reduction include:

- Nourishment is a solace cover; we use it to comfort ourselves amid stress or trouble
- Eating occupies us from sentiments of trouble, uneasiness, or anger
- Indulging greasy, sugary, or unfortunate nourishments is related to festivities and other great occasions.
- Unfortunate or sugary nourishments are a prize.
- Indulging encourages you to pack the dread that you won't have the option to get in shape.
- Nourishment is a wellspring of amusement when exhausted.

At last, accomplishing long-term weight loss requires these main drivers to be surveyed, comprehended, and reframed.

What's more, that is actually what hypnosis can enable us to accomplish.

Reframing Your Food Addiction with Hypnosis

The initial step of utilizing entrancing for weight reduction:

Identifying why you aren't accomplishing your objectives. How does this work? Regularly, a subliminal specialist will ask you inquiries identified with your weight reduction, for example, inquiries concerning your eating and exercise habits.

This information gathering recognizes what you may require help chipping away at.

You'll, at that point, be guided through acceptance, a procedure to loosen up the brain and body and go into a condition of entrancing. While in entrancing, your psyche is exceptionally suggestible.

You've shed your basic, conscious personality – and the subliminal specialist can talk straightforwardly to your unconscious thoughts.

In hypnosis, the hypnotherapist will furnish you with positive proposals, insistences and may request that you envision changes.

You can attempt it right now with our many weight loss entrancing chronicles! Positive recommendations for weight loss entrancing may include:

Improving Confidence. Positive proposals will engage your sentiments of certainty through empowering language.

You are picturing Success. During hypnosis, you might be approached to picture meeting your weight loss goals and to envision how it causes you to feel. You are reframing Your

Inner Voice. Entrancing can assist you with restraining an inward voice who "wouldn't like" to surrender unfortunate nourishments, and transform it into a partner in your weight reduction venture who's fast with positive recommendations and is progressively balanced.

You are tapping the Unconscious. In the hypnotic state, you can start to distinguish the oblivious examples that lead to undesirable eating.

You can turn out to be progressively mindful of why we are settling on undesirable nourishment decisions and bit control and build up increasingly careful procedures for settling on nourishment decisions.

They are fighting Off Fear. Hypnotic recommendations can assist you with subduing your dread of not making weight reduction progress. Fear is a No. 1 reason individuals may never begin in any case.

Distinguishing and Reframing Habit Patterns. Once in hypnosis, you can inspect and investigate ways you use eating and "turn off" these automatic reactions.

Through rehashed positive insistences, we can start to slow and eventually totally evacuate programmed, oblivious ideas.

You are growing New Coping Mechanisms.

Through entrancing, you can build up increasingly solid approaches to adapt to pressure, feelings, and connections.

For instance, you may be approached to picture an upsetting circumstance and afterward envision yourself reacting

Chapter 6

Overcome Your Weight Loss Plateau

There's no room for error when you set yourself up with strict, black and white guidelines to abstain entirely from those foods. You are on or off the diet, either. You're off the wagon once you've had the cookie - and that means anything goes.

What's the difference between two and twelve cookies? Next week you will continue the sugar ban again - or probably next month.

Here's the worst part: the guilt, embarrassment, and self-criticism resulting from "breaking the rules" that prevent you from making reasonable efforts.

It may sound like self-sabotage, but it's very logical in fact: if you realize you're punishing yourself for failure, why try? Who needs punishment? In our curriculum, we refer to ourselves as the Inner Critic, the self-critical element.

It's a cruel inner voice that focuses on only one part of ourselves—such as a sugar weakness—with a mean heart, without looking at the bigger picture of who we are.

The criticism of getting dishes from the Inner Critic causes one to feel worse and have less desire to adjust. If it's so frustrating to our accumulated experience trying to improve our actions, we stop working.

Health psychologists refer to the "abstinence violation effect" spiral of failure-shame-avoidance, which results from violating rigid rules.

Health Happens "In the Middle"

It's unusual that our days go exactly as expected – at work, at home, and anywhere in between. Our children get sick; we get sick; we get stuck in the traffic; we get bad news about the wellbeing of a friend; our supervisor adds a job to our overflowing plate.

Not only is the diet mentality detrimental to weight loss and physical wellbeing; it also runs counter to emotional health.

The word cognitive rigidity is used by psychologists to describe thought patterns that are so entrenched that people have difficulty thinking flexibly.

Humans are not robots. It's natural to have a hard time implementing a strict plan — whether it's a diet, a "detox," or an effort to give up sugar in cold-turkey. In an ever-changing environment, versatility is key to maintaining healthy eating habits.

The entire notion of versatility is frightening for many people who have struggled with their eating habits, bringing to mind an "everything goes" mindset that can do nothing but curb their unhealthy habits. And that preoccupation is correct. We don't say "anything goes."

Having plenty of freedom but no expectations or guidance can leave us wandering in our attempts to make changes — we don't even know where to begin.

How then, without being locked into a fixed program, can you make changes?

Behavior-changing progress is most successful when individuals are "in the middle" and not at the extremes. It is crucial to have goals and expectations.

However, there is still enough flexibility to allow you to adjust to changing circumstances - including getting off track - to improve your eating habits and continue those changes.

It runs counter to the mindset of the diet, and contrary to "everything goes "—and is sustainable.

Get Moving Mindfully

Like healthy food, physical activity (and its lack) plays a significant role in our general wellbeing, our risk of illness, our mental health and happiness, and our weight, of course.

But as with food, trends are troubling over the last fifty years, with more and more people living sedentary lives.

The numbers are different, but they're grim. Surveys show that just 20 percent of American adults say they follow the fitness requirements for exercise and strength training, according to the Centers for Disease Control, but the truth could be much worse.

Researchers at the National Cancer Institute, who used motion sensors to monitor people more accurately, found that only 5% had at least 30 minutes of moderate-intensity exercise most days of the week.

In January, new participants who plan to work out are filling the gym every day. In the short term, this method can be very motivating but is generally not sustainable.

Once again, it's the power-through-it approach, based on external motivation and punishment/reward (think of "no pain, no benefit" and the glistening, unattainable bodies on show in running-shoe ads).

To others, starting is too daunting, while many others start and then fizzle out. And some people are overdoing exercise, which can be as harmful as underdoing it. Both of these trends are indicators of a shifting outward-in approach.

There is a safe, middle way that begins with yourself tuning in. The why of exercise, as with food, tells them how? Tell yourself, "What motivates me to exercise? Who do I do this for? "May provide significant detail. For example, you might realize you've been jogging to keep up with (and maybe impress) your athletic sister-in-law, but you don't enjoy it—and what you love is dancing.

What if you viewed physical activity as an opportunity to help your overall wellbeing? What if you gain strength, bring joy and fun, and feel confident and competent, instead of concentrating on a specific target (losing a certain amount of weight or fitting into a certain dress), or seeing exercise as something you "should" do? What if you just did it for yourself?

Instead of concentrating on the result, you should focus on the process—miles jogged, pounds lost, calories burned. That means adapting to the way your body feels before, during, and after exercise.

That lets you stay versatile. If you know that when swimming your shoulder gets stiff, you should stop before it is an injury — and maybe change your routine to include other activities as well.

It helps to differ between a few events for most people, both to avoid damage and to keep off boredom.

If you're feeling resistant to the thought of exercise, consider why you're exercising—what you want in the long run. Rather than telling yourself, "Do I feel like doing some exercise?" Mind why this is important to you.

When done in a safe, conscientious way, exercise for a simple purpose is a positive feedback loop: it feels fantastic!

And though when you're exercising you feel any pain or exhaustion, you'll experience the benefits shortly after. In fact, with exercise, sometimes the effects are felt faster than with changes in the diet.

Our bodies and brains—all from our blood vessels and mitochondria to the feel-good neurotransmitters in our mind—function better when we frequently travel about.

It's vital for self-care and overall wellbeing to find your way to the right routine — not too little, not too much, and something you enjoy.

Positive Affirmations for Weight Loss

The only thing that is important when it comes to health and fitness is a balanced bodyweight. What decides your health is your weight! That's why, any time you go for a checkup, doctors always check your weight.

The problem today is that people do not look at weight loss as a health problem anymore, instead of considering it as more of a looks problem, which is why they don't get anywhere.

If they could only understand how important weight is to health, people would be more inspired to lose weight.

Your weight makes you who you are. Whether you like it or not, you will be judged by it; this is just part of life. In fact, in America alone, over 65% of the population is either overweight or obese.

That's two out of every three Americans. There are over 1 billion individuals worldwide that fall into this group!

That's 1 in every 7 people around the world who have weight issues! It's no wonder healthcare is such a big issue.

So, you need to lose weight quickly and lose it right away, whether you're overweight or obese, but how are you going to lose weight the best way?

The response to that is the biggest hidden weight loss mystery.

The basic fact is that individuals DON'T know how to lose weight. In hopes that it will succeed, many will only try the old eat less and exercise more theory.

Nonetheless, this mentality of weight loss is what ultimately keeps the world the same way with the same issues. People only do whatever the media and so-called experts tell them while doing the little operation. This is because there is no balance, which is why many struggle to lose weight!

The key to weight loss is balance. Every day, you need to eat the correct number of calories and exercise for the correct amount of time each week.

For overall and long-term results, getting the balance is the best way! It's so important to understand because the secret of equilibrium can go to such endless depths.

However, you need to be well informed about it and its relationship with weight loss to make use of balance.

You need to learn more about weight loss and all the elements of it. If you're serious about weight loss, then you can spend some of your time learning the secrets of weight loss.

It's not going to be that hard if you know what there is to know about it. If you want to go further into weight loss, you're going to find there's so much more to it.

Many factors have to be considered, including a good diet, weight, metabolism, and even the human body itself! To grasp weight loss entirely, there are so many things to remember.

You must first become educated about weight loss if you want to commit to it. You need to get to the point where you will be able to spot it immediately if you make a mistake, without any support from experts or professionals.

To succeed, you need to be alone.

The Question.

Imagine scaling the mountain to ask the wise man what the secret is to losing weight? As is always the case with the wise person on the mountain top, their answer is not only short and simple but also obvious and common sense.

The Reaction.

So, in response to the issue of the key to weight loss, the wise individual advises, first of all, to not gain weight.

Follow-Up Question and Reaction.

I asked the follow-up question to this one: If I knew how, O wise man, I would not have climbed the mountain.

The wise individual answers: In the first place, the way to reach weight loss is not to gain weight. Find the four keys to losing weight in order not to gain weight in the first place.

The Four Secrets

O wise man, what are the four secrets to losing weight? Again, I ask, but the wise person is somehow gone.

When I walk down the mountain, all I can think about is what the secrets are. The path down is long, giving time for the individual to think about the conversation.

Then it dawns on me that the answer has to be brief, concise, clear, common sense.

The four weight loss secrets must be:

- Eat Less
- Eat Right
- Enjoy Activity
- Enjoy Life

Hey, how real. The wise person has enabled me to find the final weight loss ties and to know that there are no magic bullets, but rather that it is the balancing act of eating and living and enjoying life.

Eat Less.

The first of the four secrets to losing weight is eating less. More easily said than done, you may say. I accept that. Portion control is the largest problem. Over the years, the portions have expanded not only in our homes but also in our restaurants and also in our plate size.

What was considered to be a normal daily portion several years ago is considered a junior portion now! Then again, who could avoid an offer and pick the bigger size, which is always only a little more pricey and enticing?

Eating less, however, is truly the first step. Just dish out a bit less. Don't go for second helpings. Do not super-size your meal. Stop clearing your plate.

Send the doggy bag along. If it's hard at first, try and try again. Try a natural appetite suppressant called hoodia, if anything else fails.

Be selective about your brand choice, however. Several labels are not pure and packed with fillers. Make sure that it is grown by an independent laboratory in South Africa and certified pure.

Eat Right.

The second of the four secrets is Eating Right. Eating right is about not just what you eat and drink, but what you eat and how you eat — it is necessary to chew enough and eat slowly.

A big issue for the overweight is eating wrong. It is worth exploring the use of a diet plan that helps you pursue a consistent approach to eating correctly.

There are numerous services on the market available and sold in hospitals, varying from low to very high rates.

Nonetheless, do not fall for the ads that announce a single strategy as the best.

The best program is the program that suits your personality and adapts to your lifestyle; the program which is most suitable for you.

This implies that you need to identify the different choices to decide the best match for you. No shortcuts and quick answers are available — no one would be overweight if it were.

Enjoy Activity.

Humans need activity. The third secret is to be occupied: play sports, walk, take the steps rather than the elevator, keep the car on the driveway and instead walk over.

It is also about taking up a hobby that will get you out and about. Many of these tasks, because we are social creatures, include engaging with others, which is also a positive thing.

Enjoy Life.

Life is perhaps the most important of the four secrets; it's all about enjoying the simple things that don't necessarily take a great deal of money, energy, or time.

This can be achieved by anyone; it is not just for the well-off. Get a good outlook and look for the brighter side.

Enjoy yourself, your family, and your friends. Enjoy what you do at work and what you do at home. Indulge yourself in hobbies. Learn new things and have an inquisitive mind, asking questions and obtaining replies. They all contribute to loving life.

The dictionary definition of an affirmation is the affirmation of which is already known. Affirmations of health are valuable tools for encouraging one's self to reach an optimal state of being. If you want to lose any kilos, weight loss claims might be very beneficial for you.

If you want to slash those extra pounds, it is the very first thing you should be doing.

Affirmations of weight loss might consist of emphasizing and agreeing to yourself that you just have to reinforce with yourself that you have to do away with it because you want to increase your weight when you are about to get tempted to eat.

It is something that will direct you not to slip back into your old habits but will instead help you move on to accomplish that objective instead.

It might be a slogan, a mantra, or whatever else you'd like to call it. To reduce your urge, the trick here is to send constructive messages to your brain.

There is more possibility for you to slim down through this. It's supposed to be something you trust and something that will keep you on track.

When you mention them in the present tense, the affirmations will be far clearer. Do not use the future tense as this just puts off what you want to do now.

It will give you a much deeper belief that you are ready and that you want to do this now if you place your affirmations in the present tense.

Right now, it's going to happen, and it's not something you're going to have to do in the future.

Your attitude and how you use your vocabulary play a very important role in your comments. According to Barbara Hoberman Levine, author of "Your Body Believes in Every Word You Say", if you want to concentrate on not doing it, the more your mind and body align to make a deliberate effort to do it.

People who want to lose weight will find a fight every day against cravings and temptations.

Here is where the allegations come in. As a personal motto, the very individual should "own" the affirmations, not borrow from anyone else. You will suggest phrases such as "I'm on the fitness track" or "I love how I feel today".

Write it out and place them in a location that is part of your everyday routine — say, your bathroom mirror — to make your affirmations even stronger. Before going to bed, read them to yourself each morning and every night.

Some psychologists also recommend that you snap your fingers and count how many snaps you made that day every time you come across a negative post. Analyze this and come up with a better, more practical affirmation.

Weight loss affirmations are just a mental roadmap for you to meet your target weight. In this pursuit, your mind and your body should be one.

One way you can condition your mind for the success of weight loss is by using positive affirmations.

What are positive affirmations?

Positive words are strong words that we repeat (either in our mind or out loud) to ourselves, and they are usually things we want to do.

They are used to stimulate our inner thoughts and to affect our behavior and the progress we make.

If you say them frequently with confidence and true conviction, then your subconscious mind will come to recognize them as genuine.

Your new positive self-image will be improved, and you will be charged with positive energy.

Your mindset, actions, and thoughts will shift and bring about a positive change until your mind begins to believe something is real.

Positive remarks can be customized to any purpose you want to reach, including losing weight.

Weight Loss Positive Affirmations

You need to use a handful of motivating weight loss phrases that will inspire you and reflect what you want to accomplish.

Here are some ideas for helpful weight loss statements:

- For me, losing weight comes easily.
- I will attain my targets for weight loss.[A79]
- Every day I lose weight.
- I love the taste of nutritious food.
- I have power over how much I eat.
- I do enjoy exercising; it makes me do feel healthy.
- I am getting fitter and stronger through exercise.
- I am cultivating more balanced eating habits all the time.
- Every day I get slimmer.
- I look and feel amazing.

Try to use optimistic phrases that work for you and that you feel comfortable with. You have to repeat them regularly (at least 3-4 times a day) and with real certainty, for them to work.

Repeat them when you wake up in the morning and the last thing before you go to bed.

Saying them out loud can be very motivational if you can get time alone. Write down your optimistic affirmations on a card and bring them around with you for an immediate boost at any time.

You might also be able to post them on your fridge, a brilliant way to make you think twice about unhealthy snacks.

How's your loss of weight going? Are you losing the weight you thought you were going to lose?

The expectations we set for losing weight often do not necessarily align with the actual act of losing weight.

It can be tempting to feel like it's pointless at times such as this, to just forget it and give up, then go back to the old way of eating.

In addition to keeping you on track with your weight loss goals, optimistic words can be incredibly helpful by inspiring you to stay on this healthy track every day.

Affirmations and visualizations are tools that are used to accomplish almost anything in life, and there is no exception when it comes to weight loss. If that is so, why do so many people insist that statements don't work?

They need to be carried out properly for them to work. Some individuals feel that they can master a specific subject simply by seeking knowledge here and there.

Quite often, to achieve success, a mastery of the subject is necessary.

The mediocre life that individuals build for themselves because of their negative thinking is a clear example of statements at work. Poor thinking plays a part in daily comments.

When you think negatively when you keep repeating, "I'm overweight, I hate the way I look, I'm never going to lose weight, it just doesn't work" etc. This is like a catch-22.

The best way to have control of your life is to turn your detrimental affirmations into constructive ones.

Note, it's not easy to do. Negative thinking is a custom, and it takes a deliberate, persistent effort to break a habit.

How to Use Affirmations and Visualizations For Successful Weight Loss.

Rule 1: never use negative phrases. Affirmations are directed towards the subconscious mind, and negative phrases are not defined by the subconscious mind.

For instance, if you say "I am no longer overweight", the subconscious mind focuses on the "overweight" aspect and ensures that you stay overweight because it sees it as something you want.

Rule 2: using the claims only in the present tense. Do not say, "With this program, I will lose weight"; instead say, "I weigh 120 pounds right now" (if your target weight is 120 pounds).

Rule 3: be insistent. Don't give up ever. Everything you have now in your life is because of years of poor thinking. It will take some time before you begin to see good things about your life, but often you will be shocked by how easily things can change.

What keeps you from reaching your weight loss target? There may be several causes and explanations, such as medicine or disease, to blame for difficulty losing unnecessary pounds.

A hormonal imbalance can interfere with weight gain fluctuations. Emotional tension and adverse thoughts can dampen your spirits and send conflicting messages to your body. Just like your goals, a negative body image and attitude may also cause your body to respond.

Using helpful weight loss tips and motivation will set you on a healthy path while melting fat cells to balance your body and mind.

Conclusion

For several distinct purposes, hypnosis is done today, something that was previously conceived of like a mystical trick, which doesn't work.

Nevertheless, looking at outcomes recorded by consumers over the years, particularly with weight loss, one can see that it is something that will help you move ahead in life.

Aside from reducing weight, when dealing with addiction, sleep loss, struggles, and more, it will help you conquer your worries, fatigue, anxiety, depression, and also support your emotional well-being.

It also helps to encourage fitness and wellbeing as a big aspect, helping you to practice mindfulness, which is something most people don't know how to do.

It serves as a psychiatric therapy and will make you experience many more rewards than you ever felt were necessary to support your well-being.

This encourages you to undergo improvements in your emotions, attitudes, beliefs, and experiences, which may be achieved either in a therapeutic environment or in the privacy of your own home.

Hypnosis has been effective in increasing deep sleep in people by up to 80%, which helps us to wake up every day more energized and renewed.

Sincerest plays such a crucial role in our daily lives and is important for our wellbeing to be maintained, it also goes to show how effective hypnosis can be.

You are most likely mindful of the amazing advantages that hypnosis for weight reduction has in store for you.

Our listed health benefits include: It helps to fix sleep habits, such as anxiety, sleepwalking, and having general difficulty sleeping, and update your mind on the advantages you might encounter from pursuing one of our hypnosis for losing weight sessions.

If you suffer from some of these symptoms, by practicing a hypnotherapy regimen every day, you will learn how to calm your subconscious and shape healthier sleeping habits.

Provided that hypnotherapy tends to solve any problems linked to insufficient sleep, it also assists the path of weight reduction, since sleep is essential to sustain a correctly healthy mind and body.

It also allows your metabolism to work properly, which allows you to lose weight, retains the cells in your body, and maintains your whole body's proper cohesive functioning. It helps to alleviate stress and anxiety.

Hypnotherapy operates by calming the mind, helping people to become in town with themselves and gain a sense of calm and confidence throughout their lives because depression and anxiety are encountered due to excess feelings and becoming excessively influenced by the everyday pressures of life.

Hypnotherapy is designed to help you to let go of any unpleasant emotions, attitudes, and common interactions that you might have, turning your attention to happier stuff.

CPSIA information can be obtained
at www.ICGtesting.com
Printed in the USA
BVHW070909150321
602550BV00011B/1355

RAPID WEIGHT LOSS HYPNOSIS

Do you want to lose weight quickly without changing your eating habits? Are you giving up and you think there's nothing you can do? To discover how to solve this problem, keep reading.

Everyone wants to change their life but they complain without doing anything about their situation. Weight loss is only possible with exercise and balanced meals, but now you can get some extra help.

Self-hypnosis appears to be a useful tool for losing weight. It helps you lose moderate amounts of weight regularly, resulting in safe and lasting weight loss. Combined with exercise it helps you get better results!

Is this book for you?
This book provides guided meditation, affirmation, and self-hypnosis scripts that will not only open your mind to bigger and better possibilities but also help you shed the unwanted pounds healthily and sustainably.

In this book you will learn:
- Applications of hypnosis
- Working with the subconscious
- Changing behavioral models
- Benefits of hypnosis
- Treatment of stress with self-hypnosis
- Weight loss through hypnosis and other techniques
- Hypnosis and weight loss
- Techniques to reach your ideal weight
- Talking into the mind of your own body
- Hypnosis session for portion management
- Mini habits for great results
- Reframing your food addiction with hypnosis
- Overcome your weight loss plateau
- Get moving mindfully
- Weight loss positive affirmations
- And much more!

Even if you have tried many diets but they did not work, with this book you can learn the best ways to burn fat quickly and naturally.

Start Your Journey To A Healthy Lifestyle!!

ISBN 978-1-80221-461-1
90000

9 781802 214611